ublished 2012 by Pearson Education Limited

hed 2014 by Routledge
Square, Milton Park, Abingdon, Oxon OX14 4RN
hird Avenue, New York, NY 10017, USA

dge is an imprint of the Taylor & Francis Group, an informa business

es

edge and best practice in this field are constantly changing. As new research and experience broaden our
standing, changes in research methods, professional practices, or medical treatment may become necessary.

titioners and researchers must always rely on their own experience and knowledge in evaluating and using any
nation, methods, compounds, or experiments described herein. In using such information or methods they should be
ul of their own safety and the safety of others, including parties for whom they have a professional responsibility.

e fullest extent of the law, neither the Publisher nor the authors, contributors, or editors, assume any liability for any
and/or damage to persons or property as a matter of products liability, negligence or otherwise, or from any use or
tion of any methods, products, instructions, or ideas contained in the material herein.

13: 978-0-273-74402-3 (hbk)

h Library Cataloguing-in-Publication Data
alogue record for this book is available from the British Library

ry of Congress Cataloging-in-Publication Data
atalog record for this book is available from the Library of Congress

set in 8/9.5pt Helvetica by 35

T0186505

contents

Aim of this recap book:

- To recap on the up-to-date guidelines set out by the Resuscitation Council 2010 on cardiopulmonary resuscitation.
- To promote good practice.
- To support nursing students in clinical placement.
- To use as an aide-memoire for Objective Structured Clinical Examinations (OSCEs).

The most life-threatening situation a student nurse could be called to is a casualty who is not breathing. Early assistance is of the utmost importance to save the life of the casualty, as brain cells that are starved of oxygen start to die within a few minutes. As a student nurse you can artificially breathe for and pump oxygen around the body until emergency help arrives. A combination of chest compressions and rescue breaths are known as cardiopulmonary resuscitation (CPR).

Up-to-date resuscitation skills and knowledge are vital for student nurses to optimise survival for the victims of cardiopulmonary arrest. The Nursing and Midwifery Council (NMC) *Code of Professional Conduct* (2008) states that as a professional, you are personally accountable for actions and omissions in your practice and must always be able to justify your decisions. The Resuscitation Council guidelines 2010 also state:

s important that those who may be present at the scene
cardiac arrest . . . should have learnt the appropriate
uscitation skills and be able to put them into practice.'

s survival guide helps guide you through the important
ctical procedures and theory required for correct
diopulmonary resuscitation (CPR) with additional advice
related procedures such as the recovery position, the
king patient and top-to-toe survey.

te: please ensure that you have had your CPR update
actical and theory) at the establishment where you are
dying, as this is only a recap book.

WHAT DO THE LETTERS CPR REPRESENT?

dio (heart)
monary (lungs)
suscitation (attempt to restart the heart)

Cardiovascular System – Anatomy and Physiolo

To understand the theory behind the procedure of cardiopulmona resuscitation you need to understand the anatomy and physiology of the cardiovascular system (see Figure 1).

Figure 1   The structure of the heart

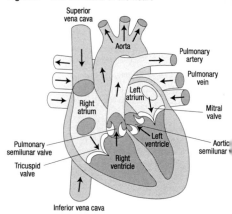

Inferior vena cava

Activity: See if you can revise the structure of the heart a its functions to help you understand how cardiopulmonary resuscitation works, using Figure 1 above and referring to your anatomy and physiology book.

■ THE FUNCTION OF THE HEART

The heart acts as a pump that pushes blood around the bo by rhythmic contractions. Blood vessels act as a vehicle,

rying the blood around the body (see Figure 2). The term
rdiac is a term used in relation to the heart.

ure 2 The circulatory pathway

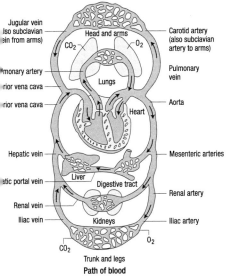

Jugular vein
lso subclavian
ein from arms)

Head and arms

CO_2

O_2

Carotid artery
(also subclavian
artery to arms)

monary artery

Pulmonary
vein

Lungs

rior vena cava

rior vena cava

Heart

Aorta

Hepatic vein

Mesenteric arteries

atic portal vein

Liver

Digestive tract

Renal vein

Renal artery

Iliac vein

Kidneys

Iliac artery

CO_2

O_2

Trunk and legs
Path of blood

The cycle begins in the right atrium, where the blood flows
through a valve called the **tricuspid**, to the **right ventricle**.
From the right ventricle the blood is pumped out to
the **pulmonary semilunar valve** and travels through the
ulmonary artery to the lungs.

- From the lungs, blood flows back through the **pulmonary vein** to the left atrium.
- The blood travels through a valve called the **mitral valve** to the **left ventricle**, and is then pumped through the **aortic semilunar** valve to the **aorta**.
- The **aorta** divides and the blood is shared between major arteries which supply the upper and lower body parts.
- The blood travels in the **arteries** to the smaller **arterioles** then to the **capillaries** which provide nutrition to each cell.
- The deoxygenated blood travels to the **venules**, which lead into veins, to the **inferior and superior vena cava.**
- The final stage is where the blood travels back to the **right atrium** where the process begins all over again.

Source: Waugh and Grant (2006)

Basic life support guidelines (out of hospital)

■ STEP 1: APPROACHING THE CASUALTY

Firstly, always check the area for any signs of danger before approaching the casualty. There is no point in endangering yourself and adding to the casualties. See Figure 3.

Figure 3 A few examples of danger

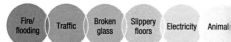

Tip When checking the area for signs of danger you must always approach the casualty with caution: he/she might be pretending to have collapsed in order to initiate an attack

STEP 2: SHAKE AND SHOUT

en the area is safe, attend to the casualty by kneeling
their side and shaking their shoulders, at the same time
uting in their ear, 'Are you alright?' If there is more than
casualty, prioritise the care for casualties involved, for
mple: a patient who has no signs of life will need immediate
ntion, rather than a casualty who has a graze on the hand.

*Make sure you talk to them close to their ear and not too far
away, as they may be semi-conscious and not hear you!*

e patient responds to your call, then continue to perform
p-to-toe assessment of the casualty and then place the
ualty in the recovery position (this will be explained later,
below).

Reassess the casualty continually until emergency help arrives.

STEP 3: IF THE CASUALTY DOES NOT RESPOND TO YOUR COMMAND

ossible turn the casualty on his/her back, firstly check the
vay, and look into the casualty's mouth to see whether
e is any obstruction. If there is an object close to the front
he mouth you may try to remove it, but if it is further back
should leave the object in place as you may be at risk of
hing it further down or the casualty may bite down on
r fingers.

Then **look, listen and feel** for signs of life for 10 seconds!
this by firstly placing one hand on the casualty's forehead
place the finger tips from the other hand under the
ualty's chin. Tilt the forehead and chin backwards, to
n up the airway.

This is known as 'head tilt – chin lift'.

- **Look** – for signs of life. Observe the patient's condit and chest rising.
- **Listen** – for signs of life. Listen for breath sounds.
- **Feel** – for the casualty's breath on your cheek.

Tip 'Agonal' breathing – this is when the casualty is taking gas of breath before breathing ceases: **this breathing is not normal!** and is a sign for starting CPR.

■ STEP 4: CALL FOR HELP AND ASK FOR AN AUTOMAT DEFIBRILLATOR (AED)

Call for help. The sooner help arrives, the sooner the casua can be treated by the emergency services. A bystander ma ring for an ambulance! But remember, do not leave the casualty unless it is necessary!

The person who phones the emergency services (999) should clearly state the following:

- Address of where the casualty is or landmark.
- How many casualties there are.
- What appears to have happened, including the casualty condition.
- Age and sex of casualty.
- First aid already carried out.
- A contact number.

Tip An AED is an automated defibrillator, a machine that helps the heart to restart and the patient to resume breathing. The AED can be found in some public places and gives clea simple instructions on how to use it.

Electrical defibrillation (AED) is well established as the only effective therapy for cardiac arrest caused by ventricular fibrillation or pulseless ventricular tachycardia (Resuscitati Council 2010). See Figure 4 overleaf.

Figure 4 AED algorithm

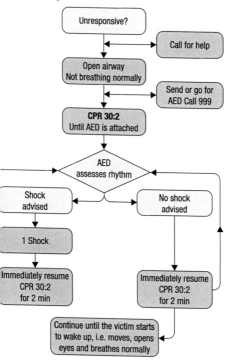

Source: Resuscitation Council (UK) (2010) *Resuscitation Guidelines 2010*. London, Resuscitation Council (UK). Reproduced with kind permission

■ STEP 5: NO SIGNS OF LIFE (NO CARDIAC OR RESPIRATORY OUTPUT): COMMENCE CHEST COMPRESSIONS

Kneel by the side of the casualty and open the casualty's clothing to view the chest.

Begin chest compressions (**immediately**) by placing on hand on the centre of the casualty's chest (inter-nipple line using the heel of the hand only.

Tip *The centre of the chest is the lower half of the sternum.*

Take the other hand and place it on top of the hand that is placed on the centre of the casualty's chest. The fingers should be interlocked as in the figure.

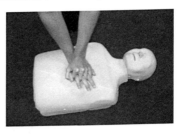

Tip *No pressure should be applied to:*
- *the upper abdomen.*
- *the bottom end of the sternum.*

Press down on the chest 5–6 cm in depth (100–120 times per minute) without removing your hands from the chest.

nt 30 of these without stopping and then stop! Administer
rescue breaths.

*Ensure that for compressions your arms are kept straight
and that your body is vertically positioned over the casualty's
chest. Compression and release should take the same
amount of time.*

STEP 6: RESCUE BREATHS

Figure 5 opposite.

the head tilt–chin lift procedure to open up the casualty's
way.

ch the soft part of the casualty's nose closed, letting the
uth stay open.

e a breath in yourself, and then cover the casualty's
uth with your mouth, ensuring there is no air escaping
ating a good seal).

w into the casualty's mouth, looking for the casualty's
st rising.

e your mouth away and watch the chest fall.

eat the rescue breath again.

*This should take no more than five seconds, but it should
take one second to make the chest rise (this is how normal
breathing works).*

Figure 5   Rescue breaths

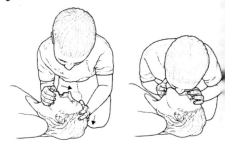

Repeat this cycle: 30 chest compressions / 2 rescue breaths (30:2), until emergency help arrives, stopping only if you're too tired to continue or the casualty starts breathing. Otherwise: do not stop the sequence of 30 ches compressions and 2 rescue breaths!

Tip   Be continually aware of a change in the casualty's conditio for example regaining consciousness.

the rescue breaths sequence does not show the chest rising and falling:

Look in the casualty's mouth for any signs of obstruction, for example food or foreign object. An obstruction can block the airway and stop the casualty breathing. If any obstruction is present and **visible**, remove it if it is at the front of the mouth and obtainable, if it is further back leave it in place rather than take the risk of pushing it further back into the airway.

Check that the head is positioned far enough back and the chin is tilted sufficiently.

Continue with 30 chest compressions : 2 rescue breaths.

If you are not alone, take it in turns to perform CPR (change over every 1–2 minutes, to prevent one person becoming too tired). If you are unwilling to perform rescue breaths, perform chest compressions only, at a continuous rate of 100–120 min. Only stop if the casualty shows signs of life!

STEP 7: MOUTH-TO-NOSE VENTILATION (ALTERNATIVE TO MOUTH-TO-MOUTH)

This may be used if a patient has received trauma to the mouth internally and/or externally. See Figure 6 overleaf. Those with a 'duty of care' should be taught chest compressions and rescue breaths (Resuscitation Council, 2010).

Figure 6 Adult Basic Life Support

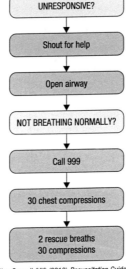

Source: Resuscitation Council (UK) (2010) *Resuscitation Guidelines 2010*. Lond
Resuscitation Council (UK). Reproduced with kind permission

suscitation in hospital

he case of an arrest occurring in a clinical area, the
owing points should be remembered:

The main aim of in-hospital resuscitation is to recognise
cardiac arrest immediately.

The person calling the arrest team would dial 2222 from
the clinical placement phone.

Instead of mouth-to-mouth (two rescue breaths) an oxygen
mask attached to an ambulatory bag will administer 100%
oxygen to the patient (see Figure 7). The ambulatory bag
will be squeezed twice to replicate two breaths.

Defibrillation is attempted within three minutes.

*Tracheal intubation should only be performed by individuals
who are trained in using this equipment.*

ure 7 Using an oxygen mask

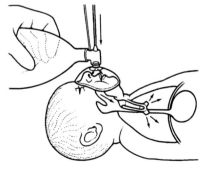

5. The emergency team will use the following equipment:
   - Defibrillator
   - CPR cart containing all equipment required in a cardiac arrest
   - CPR drug box
   - ECG machine
   - Intravenous fluid and drip stand.

The ABCDE approach referred to in Figures 8 and 9 (following) is as follows:

Airway – Is there an obstruction in the patient's mouth?

Breathing – Is the patient breathing? Look, listen, feel.

Circulation – Look at the patient's hands, are they pink or blue, do they feel warm or cold? (If the hands are cold and discoloured this could be an indication they have poor circulation.) Feel for a pulse.

Disability – Review current medication sheet to see whether it may be drug-induced; check pupil response to light, and glucose levels to ensure patient not having uncontrolled diabetes, e.g. diabetic coma.

Exposure – Removing patient's clothing, maintaining patient dignity at all times, in order to observe any injuries.

Once the cardiac arrest team arrive at the scene the Advanced Life Support procedure will be followed.

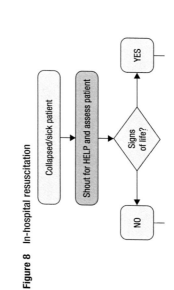

Figure 8 In-hospital resuscitation

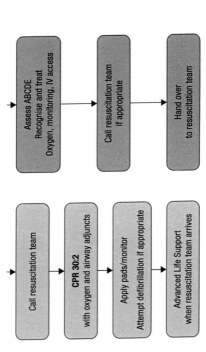

Assess ABCDE
Recognise and treat
Oxygen, monitoring, IV access

Call resuscitation team
if appropriate

Hand over
to resuscitation team

Call resuscitation team

CPR 30:2
with oxygen and airway adjuncts

Apply pads/monitor
Attempt defibrillation if appropriate

Advanced Life Support
when resuscitation team arrives

Source: Resuscitation Council (UK) (2010) *Resuscitation Guidelines 2010*. London, Resuscitation Council (UK). Reproduced with kind permission

Figure 3 Adult advanced life support

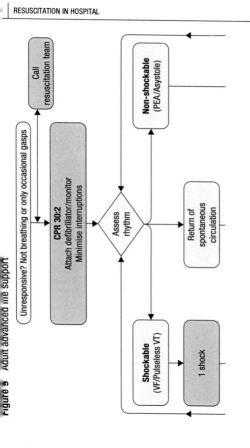

Immediately resume CPR for 2 min
Minimise interruptions

Immediately resume CPR for 2 min
Minimise interruptions

Immediate post-cardiac arrest treatment

- Use ABCDE approach
- Controlled oxygenation and ventilation
- 12-lead ECG
- Treat precipitating cause
- Temperature control/therapeutic hypothermia

During CPR

- Ensure high-quality CPR: rate, depth, recoil
- Plan actions before interrupting CPR
- Give oxygen
- Consider advanced airway and capnography
- Continuous chest compressions when advanced airway in place
- Vascular access (intravenous, intraosseous)
- Give adrenaline every 3–5 min
- Correct reversible causes

Reversible causes

- Hypoxia
- Hypovolaemia
- Hypo-/hyperkalaemia/metabolic
- Hypothermia
- Thrombosis – coronary or pulmonary
- Tamponade – cardiac
- Toxins
- Tension pneumothorax

Source: Resuscitation Council (UK) (2010) *Resuscitation Guidelines 2010.* London, Resuscitation Council (UK). Reproduced with

cisions on DNAR (Do not attempt resuscitation)

emergency medical team are responsible for making the sion whether or not to resuscitate an individual.

DNAR order can be considered if:

The patient refuses to be resuscitated should the event happen.

The patient will not survive a cardiac arrest even if CPR is attempted.

decision-making process should be based on the current delines from the BMA (2001), Resuscitation Council (UK) Royal College of Nursing (RCN) (2001). A standardised n should be used.

ection control/hand washing

ny lives are lost every year because of the spread of ctions both in hospitals and the community setting. lth care workers can take steps to prevent this through ular hand washing, as it remains the most effective way prevent the spread of infection.

CPR is an emergency; hands cannot be washed prior he procedure, but hands must be washed after the cedure.

When washing your hands always use the eight-step hand washing technique as shown in Figure 10 (based upon Ayliffe et al. 2000).

Figure 10   Hand Decontamination Technique

Decontaminate hands using soap and water using the
following eight steps. Each step consists of five strokes rubbing
backwards and forwards.

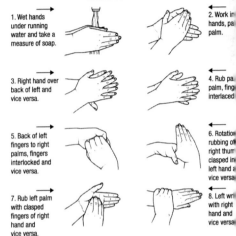

1. Wet hands under running water and take a measure of soap.

2. Work in hands, pa palm.

3. Right hand over back of left and vice versa.

4. Rub pa palm, fing interlaced

5. Back of left fingers to right palms, fingers interlocked and vice versa.

6. Rotation rubbing of right thum clasped in left hand a vice versa

7. Rub left palm with clasped fingers of right hand and vice versa.

8. Left wri with right hand and vice versa

*When using soap and water ensure hands are
thoroughly dry before continuing any task*

Now that you have the knowledge on the procedure of CPF
the next chapter will cover an example of a casualty who i
breathing.

enario 1 (patient breathing)

OAD TRAFFIC ACCIDENT

are driving along the motorway when traffic begins to
w down. Ahead you notice a collision has taken place.
 go over to offer assistance, where you are faced with a
man (casualty) lying on the road: she does appear to be
scious, but is not moving (see Figure 11 on page 31).

ion to be taken

Assess the situation, think about what you are dealing
vith, and call for help!

Make the area as safe as possible, for example if there is
 danger from traffic.

ssess all casualties if there are more than one, and give
emergency aid. It is important that you prioritise care:
vho is at most risk and who is at least risk?

 also Scenario 2 below, on dealing with more than one
ualty.

When dealing with a casualty who has been involved
 traffic accident and is breathing it is important to
ember not to move him/her until a full top-to-toe
essment has been undertaken as there may be serious
ries which cannot be seen immediately. After emergency
 has been given to the casualty you may then carry out
 top-to-toe examination; this can be done even if the
ualty is in the recovery position.

■ TOP-TO-TOE ASSESSMENT FROM A NURSING STUDENT'S POINT OF VIEW

When carrying out a top-to-toe assessment ensure that you wear gloves to protect yourself from bodily fluids, for example blood. Gently feel each area, bringing your hands out to the side to check for any blood on your gloves.

Top-to-toe assessment

AREA	SYMPTOMS	INDICATION
Head (skull and scalp)	Check for: • Swelling to the head area • Bleeding from the head area • Depression/indentations to the head soft areas	This may indicate the following: • Head injury • Fractured skull
Both ears	• Speak to the casualty; if they respond to your voice, the casualty can hear you. • Look for any blood/clear/straw-coloured fluid draining from the ears.	This may indicate: • Head injury • Fractured skull

EA	SYMPTOMS	INDICATION
th es	Now look at the pupils: • What size are the pupils? Are the pupils equal in size, or unequal? • Do the pupils react to light? If you have a pen torch you could use it to check the pupil reaction. • Are there any foreign objects in the eye? • Is there any blood in the eyes? • Is there any bruising in the whites of the eyes?	Another indication of head injury or trauma.
se	• Look for blood/clear liquid from either nostril. • Is the nose displaced?	• Possibility of head injury. • The nose may be fractured.
outh/ eth	Smell the casualty's breath. Is there any odour? For example a pear-drop smell (sugar) or alcohol. Look inside the mouth: • Are there any loose teeth/bleeding? Examine the lips: • Are the lips bleeding and are they intact?	This may indicate that the casualty is diabetic. The accident may be alcohol-induced. • This may indicate trauma to the mouth.

AREA	SYMPTOMS	INDICATION
Face	Note the colour of the face: • Is the face a pale colour, cold and clammy? • Is the face red in colour and hot to touch?	• Possible indication that the casualty is in shock. • This may indicate that the casualty has a high temperature
Neck	• Loosen the casualty's clothing so that you can observe the neck area. • Look for warning medallion. • Is there a hole in the wind pipe? • Run fingers along the spine from the base of the skull for irregularities/ tenderness.	• This will aler you that the casualty is ▮ example a diabetic or h an allergy. • This may be a new hole the casualty could have a tracheotomy

EA	SYMPTOMS	INDICATION
llar ne	Feel for any deformity, irregularities or tenderness.	
est	Ask casualty to breathe in and out: • Does the chest expand evenly, easily and equally?	• Only one side of chest rising may be an indication of a pneumothorax. • Spinal cord injury?
	• Do not move casualty to examine spine – place hand under hollow of back and feel gently for swelling and tenderness. • Examine the ribcage for any deformities. • Is there any tenderness? • Is there a grating sensation on breathing? • Is there any pain or discomfort on breathing? • Is there any sign of bleeding? • Record rate, depth and nature of breathing	• The ribs may be fractured. • By measuring the breathing a baseline observation can be identified.

AREA	SYMPTOMS	INDICATION
Both arms	<ul><li>Check movement of both arms.</li><li>Check movement of both elbows.</li><li>Check movement of both wrists.</li><li>Ask the casualty to bend and straighten fingers and to bend and straighten joints.</li><li>Can they feel normally with their fingers?</li><li>Are there any abnormal sensations?</li><li>What is the colour of the fingers – are they cyanosed (blue)?</li><li>Check for needle marks</li><li>Measure the radial pulse at the wrist</li></ul>	<ul><li>If the casual... is unable to move arms/ elbows/wris... this may indicate a fracture/spra... or strain.</li><li>Possibility o... spinal injury... nerve dama...</li><li>If the finger... are cyanose... it may relate... hypothermia... poor circulati...</li><li>This may indicate dru... abuse.</li><li>A baseline observation is essential so that a comparison can be mad... when furthe... observations are performe...</li></ul>

EA	SYMPTOMS	INDICATION
domen	Feel for tenderness/bleeding and rigidity	Internal injuries
vis	Feel both sides of hips and gently move pelvis for signs of a fracture. • Any incontinence • Bleeding from orifices	This may indicate fractured hip/pelvis.
th legs	• Signs of impaired movement/loss of sensation. • Bleeding, deformity or tenderness. Raise legs in turn, move ankles and knees	• Possibility of a fracture/ cerebral vascular accident. • If one leg appears shorter, this may suggest a hip fracture.
th feet	Check movement and feeling in all toes.	Broken toes.

ember

n contacting the emergency services you need to give
n the following information over the phone:
ocation of the accident.
lature of the accident, and whether the casualty is responsive.
Vho you are.
is accurate as you can as they may only send a car,
reas an ambulance/crew may be required (advanced life
port equipment).

Scenario 2 – Prioritising the care of several casualties

It is important that you understand you may come across a[n] accident with more than one casualty. Figure 11 is an exampl[e] of how you would prioritise the care of these casualties.

■ ROAD TRAFFIC ACCIDENT: A COLLISION HAS TAKEN PLACE INVOLVING TWO MOTORISTS AND A CYCLIST

Figure 11   Prioritisation

Casualty A:	PRIORITY: 1st
The cyclist who has been hit by a car. Lying on the road and is unconscious and not breathing.	Ensure an ambulance has been called and commence CPR

Casualty B:	PRIORITY: 2nd
The motorist who had severe impact on collision, driver still inside the car wreckage appears conscious and responsive however appears to have sustained a head injury.	Casualty breathing, awai[t] ambulance ask a member [of] the public to stay with him/[her] and monitor any changes [as] the head injury may be sev[ere] and the casualty may deteriorate rapidly

Casualty C:	PRIORITY: 3rd
The motorist with minimal impact on collision is out of the vehicle and appears to be alert however is shocked and upset on the side of the road.	Offer reassurance once th[e] other casualties have bee[n] seen to. Ask a member o[f] the public to stay with him/her

If you are faced with a situation where there is more than one casualty, always help the casualty who is not responsive as the casualty who responds is obviously alive.

·way obstruction – choking adult

·king is the physiological response to sudden airway ·truction. When you come across a casualty who is ·king you have to assess the severity of the situation ·e Figure 12) and take the appropriate action, and this will ·end on whether the casualty has a mild or severe airway ·truction.

·ure 12 Adult choking treatment algorithm

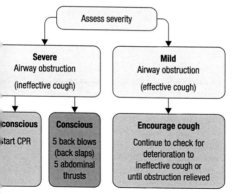

·e: Resuscitation Council (UK) (2010) *Resuscitation Guidelines 2010*, London, ·scitation Council (UK). Reproduced with kind permission

■ MILD AIRWAY OBSTRUCTION

Clinical signs: casualty breathing and responsive to questions.

The casualty may start to panic; try to keep them calm.

In this situation the casualty's airway is only partially obstructed, so encourage him/her to cough; this should be effective enough to dislodge the foreign body. If this action fails, however, the casualty may go on to develop a severe obstruction, in which case follow the steps set out below.

■ SEVERE OBSTRUCTION (PATIENT CONSCIOUS)

Clinical signs: casualty unable to speak, gasping for breath, discolouration of face.

Coughing has now become ineffective. You must immedia give five effective back slaps using the correct procedure, as follows.

Procedure for giving back slaps

1. Check the airway to ensure the foreign body has not become dislodged.
2. Position yourself to the side and slightly behind the casualty, allowing you to come close to him/her.
3. Place one hand around the casualty in order to support the chest, lean the casualty forward so that once the foreign body is dislodged it will be expelled safely.
4. Commence back slaps. Raise your free hand in the air, and using the heel of your hand give up to five sharp blows between the shoulder blades (scapulae). No more than five back slaps to be given.

It is important to assess the casualty in between each blow to ensure the foreign object has not already become expelled. If the object becomes expelled before all five back slaps have been delivered, no further back slaps are required.

ne event that the back slaps are ineffective and the airway ains obstructed, you must immediately commence ominal thrusts using the correct procedure, as follows.

e: you must have attended appropriate training to ertake this procedure.

cedure for abdominal thrusts

Stand behind the casualty placing your arms around the pper part of the abdomen. Ensure you have a firm grip. Lean the casualty forward so once the foreign body is dislodged it will be expelled safely and not remain in the airway.

Clench the fist of one hand and place it between the navel (umbilicus) and the bottom of the sternum (breastbone), grasp this hand with your other hand and pull sharply nwards and upwards.

This can be repeated up to five times.

Assess the casualty in between each abdominal thrust to ensure the foreign object has not already become expelled. DO NOT continue abdominal thrusts if object has been expelled before five thrusts have been completed.

e abdominal thrusts are not effective, check the ualty's airway; if the airway remains severely obstructed may begin the cycle of five back slaps followed by abdominal thrusts, continuing this in a cycle of three l the foreign object becomes dislodged.

■ SEVERE OBSTRUCTION (PATIENT UNCONSCIOUS)

If the client has an obstruction that can be visibly removed then the nurse can sweep it out. If the obstruction is unobtainal then the choking diagram (see p. 32) has to be addressed.

If the client has no cardiac output CPR must be commenced first.

In some cases the casualty may become unconscious, stop breathing and have no cardiac output! In this situation it is important firstly to ensure the patient is **safe, shout fo help** and **call 999** if the patient has stopped breathing and has no cardiac output.

Commence the CPR cycle until the ambulance arriv

■ RECOVERY POSITION

Once you have identified a casualty is unconscious but still breathing and a top-to-toe assessment has been made, yo would then put them into the 'recovery position'. This is a position we place patients in, in order to maintain their airway when they are breathing normally but unconscious, and in which they can recover.

Placing patient in recovery position (talk to your casua as you are following this procedure)

- Firstly gently pat down both sides of the casualty to ens there is nothing sharp in their pockets which could potentially cause further injury. If you identify somethin sharp, remove it slowly if safe to do so.
- Check the environment for danger, e.g. broken glass, spillages, etc.
- Once this has been completed the casualty may be put into the recovery position.

tly kneel down beside the casualty so you are close
ugh to manoeuvre him/her into the recovery position.
nove any article that may injure the casualty once they
e been turned over, for example: spectacles, rings.
the casualty's arm nearest to you out straight.

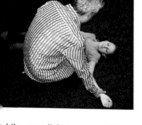

d the casualty's arm nearest to you at the elbow, and
ure the casualty's hand is pointing upwards.

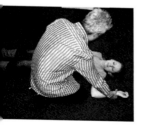

Holding the other hand (palm to palm) gently bring the casualty's hand across the chest and place the back of the hand against their opposite cheek (side nearest to the floor)

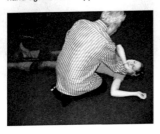

Keep your hand on the casualty's hand that is on their chest. Using your other hand bend the casualty's leg furthest away from you at the knee, and place the foot flat on the ground

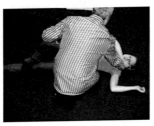

ping your hand on the casualty's knee and your palm
inst the casualty's palm (to protect their face when
ng) slowly roll the casualty towards you.

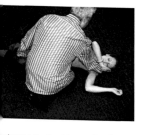

wly rest the bent leg on the floor so as not to cause any
tion and optimise comfort.

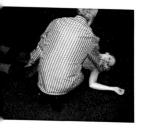

Finally ensure the airway is opened by gently tilting the he back and opening the mouth.

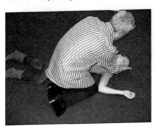

Once the casualty is in the recovery position, check that he is on its way, and if not, send help to call for an ambulanc Monitor breathing or any sudden changes in condition.

Tip *If the casualty is in this position for a prolonged period of t there is an increased risk of pressure ulcer development. I therefore important to ensure that the position of the casua is changed every 30 minutes to minimise this risk.*

Recap quiz

1. What does CPR stand for?
2. What would you understand an unsafe environment to mean?
3. Where should you touch a casualty to assess whether they are responsive?
4. What signs of life are you looking for?
5. How do you check for breathing?

How do you place a casualty in the recovery position?

If someone has a mild airway obstruction, what action would you take?

If you come across someone with a severe airway obstruction, what action would you take?

How do you open an airway?

If a casualty is not breathing, what should you do next?

Where would you place your hands during chest compressions?

What is commenced after compressions?

What is the ratio in which you continue CPR?

Practice the recovery position with a partner.

enario 3 – in community (patient not breathing)

■ are walking along the high street late at night ■owing a shift at work. You notice a man (casualty) ■g on the ground; on approaching him it appears ■s unresponsive. A crowd has begun to gather.

■ECAP QUESTIONS

■ions: Put the following procedure in the correct sequence ■ 1–12. Check your answer at the end of this booklet.

■hout for help and the automatic defibrillator (AED).

■heck in the patient's mouth to see if there is any object ■tuck, blocking the airway. If there is an object in the patient's ■nouth and it is near to their teeth within easy reach you may ■■e able to remove it. However it is important to remember ■hat if the object is further down, you should **NOT** attempt to ■emove it as you could be pushing it down even further. You ■re also at risk of the patient biting down on your fingers.

- Once you have established the casualty is unresponsive shout for help and ask a lay person to call for an ambulance (999).
- If the object cannot be removed you can still continue with the CPR cycle.
- Firstly approach the casualty, gently tap them on the shoulder and ask them if they can hear you.
- 30 chest compressions of adequate force and depth at a rate of 120 per minute and 5–6 cm in depth.
- Check the casualty's breathing and circulation; placing one hand on the forehead and placing two fingers gently under the chin, tilt the casualty's head back. Lower your ear to the casualty's mouth and feel for any breath on your cheek. At the same time look down the body at the casualty's chest to see whether it is rising and falling. You will need to do this for 10 seconds. Once you have established the patient is not breathing, you must commence the CPR cycle.
- Commence CPR by interlocking both hands one on top of the other, place the heel of the hand underneath in the middle of the chest (between the nipples) and commence compressions.
- Check the area for danger.
- Continue this at a ratio of 30:2. You must continue until the ambulance crew arrives, or you feel unable to carry on, or the casualty starts to breathe again.
- After 30 compressions proceed straight to two mouth-to-mouth ventilations (rescue breaths). Use one hand on the forehead to gently tilt the casualty's head back (opening up the airway), and pinch the casualty's nose. Place your mouth over the casualty's mouth, ensuring that you ma

good seal (no air can escape from the sides of the
mouth). Give two rescue breaths.

As you are giving each breath, look along the chest wall
or chest expansion to ensure breaths are effective.

Scenario 4 – Basic life support in hospital
(patient shows no sign of life)

----

are a student nurse on placement and in handover you
told that Mr Sam Brown's condition has deteriorated and
or resuscitation. Whilst going around to say good morning
the patients you approach Mr Brown, who appears
responsive. What would you do?

RECAP QUESTIONS – CHOOSE THE CORRECT
ACTION FOR EACH

How do you check whether the patient is responsive or not?

a) Shake and shout, 'Hello, can you hear me?'
b) Shake
c) Shout 'Hello, can you hear me?'

You look in the patient's mouth and see that he has a
piece of bread from breakfast hanging out of his mouth.
What would you do?

a) Leave it there?
b) Remove it if the bread is near to the front of the mouth.
c) Push it back in the mouth.

You look, listen and feel for the patient's breath sounds,
for how long?

a) 3 minutes
b) 1 minute
c) 10 seconds

4. Mr Brown shows no sign of life: what would you do next?
   a) Pull the emergency bell, ask somebody to call 2222, lay the patient flat and commence CPR.
   b) Go and get help.
   c) Start compressions, ask somebody to call 2222, pull the patient flat.

5. How many compressions to breaths do you commence for Mr Brown?
   a) 20
   b) 40
   c) 30

6. A facial mask and ambulatory bag will be attached to an oxygen supply to administer two rescue breaths to Mr Brown. How much oxygen will be attached to the facial mask?
   a) 20%
   b) 12%
   c) 100%

7. What equipment will the emergency team bring with the to Mr Brown's bedside?
   a) Bandages, sling, medication
   b) ECG machine, CPR drugs, defibrillator, intravenous fluids, blood pressure machine
   c) ECG machine, tympanic thermometer

8. What would you do if you had started chest compressio on Mr Brown and you felt very tired?
   a) Continue and struggle.
   b) Stop and go and do something else.
   c) Ask somebody to take over immediately so that CPR continues.

ash trolley

rash trolley (see Figure) has all the required equipment
a sudden cardiac arrest/emergency situation. The trolley
uld be checked during each shift using a checklist:
will ensure that the trolley is regularly stocked and
dy for use. It will also need to be restocked after use
n emergency situation.

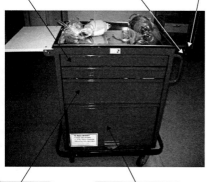

ugs required e.g.
adrenaline 1 mg
niodarone 300mg

Portable oxygen
and suction

Defibrillator

way equipment
. pocket mask,
ropharyngeal
airway

Circulation equipment,
e.g. Hartmann's solution,
sodium chloride

Airway equipment

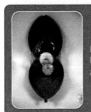

Pocket mask
Used during CPR for ventilations
and oxygen delivery

AmbiBag and mask
Used in hospital for ventilations
and delivery of oxygen

Endotracheal tube, used to
open the airway and
promote lung ventilation

Oropharyngeal airway sizes 2, 3, 4
Maintains the oral airway, can be
used for suctioning

way equipment continued

Laryngoscope is used to insert laryngeal mask airway and endotracheal intubation tube

Nasopharyngeal airway Maintains the nasal airway; can be used for suctioning

Laryngeal mask airways, size 4, 5 Maintains an airway, sits on the larynx, usually used during theatre

Magill forceps Used to remove objects lodged in the mouth

Recap quiz: answers

1. Cardiopulmonary resuscitation
2. Broken glass, spillages, traffic, wires, electricity, etc.
3. On the shoulders
4. Breathing, movement, response
5. Look, listen and feel for 10 seconds
6. Recovery position (see description earlier in text)

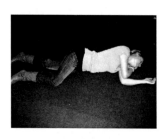

7. Encourage to cough
8. Give five effective back slaps; if ineffective give five abdominal thrusts (cycle of 3)
9. Head tilt, chin lift
10. Call an ambulance, or 2222 if in a hospital environme
11. Centre of the chest in between the nipples
12. Two effective breaths
13. 30:2 (30 compressions, 2 breaths)

enario 3: answers

Check the area for danger.

Firstly approach the casualty, gently tap them on the shoulder and ask them if they can hear you.

Once you have established the casualty is unresponsive, shout for help (999) and ask a lay person to call for an ambulance (999).

Check in the patient's mouth to see if there is any object stuck, blocking the airway. If there is an object in the patient's mouth and it is near to their teeth within easy reach you may be able to remove it. However, it is important to remember that if the object is further down you do **NOT** attempt to remove it as it could be pushed down even further. You are also at risk of the patient biting down on your fingers.

If the object cannot be removed, you can still continue with the CPR cycle.

Check the casualty's breathing and circulation; placing one hand on the forehead and placing two fingers gently under the chin, tilt the casualty's head back. Lower your ear to the casualty's mouth and feel for any breath on your cheek. At the same time look down the body at the casualty's chest to see whether it is rising and falling. You will need to do this for 10 seconds. Once you have established the patient is not breathing, you must commence the CPR cycle.

Shout for help and the automated defibrillator (AED). Commence CPR by interlocking both hands one on top of the other; using the heel of the hand underneath, place it in the middle of the chest (between the nipple and commence compressions.

9. Thirty chest compressions of adequate force and dept at a rate of 120 per minute and 5–6 cm in depth.

10. After 30 compressions proceed straight to two mouth-to-mouth ventilations (rescue breaths). Using one hand on the forehead, gently tilt the casualty's head back (opening up the airway) and pinch the casualty's nose. Place your mouth over the casualty's mouth, ensuring that you make a good seal (no air ca escape from the sides of the mouth). Give two rescue breaths.

11. As you are giving each breath, look along the chest w for chest expansion to ensure breaths are effective.

12. Continue this at a ratio of 30:2 until the ambulance cr arrives, or you feel unable to carry on, or the casualty starts to breathe again.

Scenario 4: answers

1. a) Shake and shout, 'Hello, can you hear me?'
2. b) Remove it if the bread is near to the front of the mou
3. c) 10 seconds.
4. a) Pull the emergency bell, ask somebody to call 2222, lay the patient flat and commence CPR.
5. c) 30.
6. c) 100%.
7. b) ECG machine, CPR drugs, defibrillator, intravenous fluids, blood pressure machine.
8. c) Ask somebody to take over immediately so that CPR continues.

erences

fe, G. A. J., Lowbury, E. J. L., Geddes, A. M. and
Villiams, J. D. (2000) *Control of Hospital Infection:
A Practical Handbook*, 4th edn, London, Arnold.

sing and Midwifery Council (2008) *Code of Professional
Conduct: Standards for Conduct, Performance and Ethics*,
London, NMC.

uscitation Council (UK) (2010) *Resuscitation Guidelines
2010*. London, Resuscitation Council (UK).

ugh, A. and Grant, A. (2006) *Ross and Wilson Anatomy
and Physiology in Health and Illness*, 10th edn, Edinburgh,
Churchill Livingstone.

eful websites

www.bma.org.uk
www.redcross.org.uk
www.nmc-uk.org
www.doh.gov.uk
www.nice.org.uk
www.bhf.org.uk
www.rcn.org.uk
www.resus.org.uk

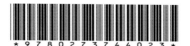

T - #0001 - 071024 - C0 - 120/80/3 - SB - 9780273744023 - Gloss Laminatio